To the dentists who put
smiles on kids ' faces all around the world

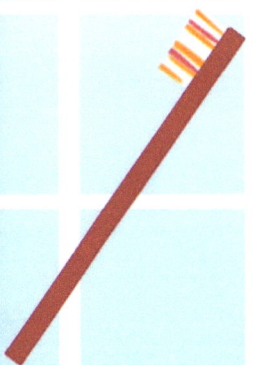

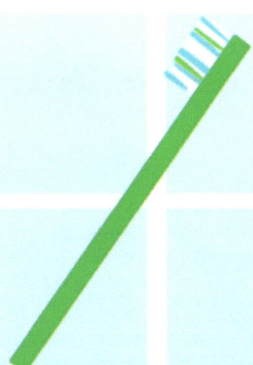

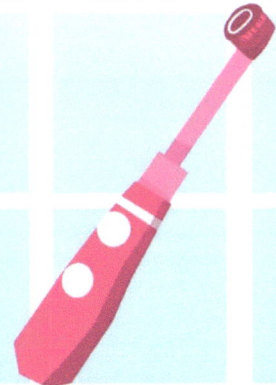

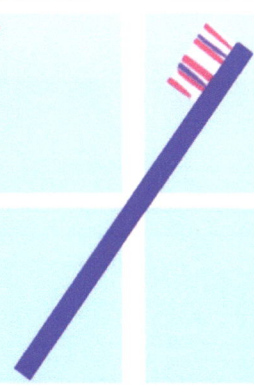

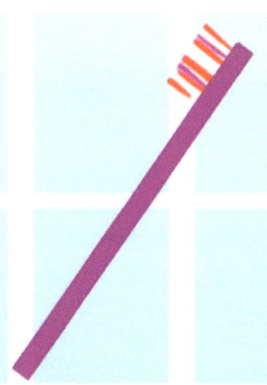

The main character of this book is based on the real-life personality of Samia Ali from
Samia's Life

For information contact:
Samia's Life at www.samiaslife.com

Written and designed by Dr. Cymanthia Connell and Adam Ali
ISBN: Hardcopy   978-1-7346872-1-7
         Paperback   978-1-7346872-2-4
         Ebook   978-1-7346872-0-0

Library of Congress Control Number: 2020908658

Published by Cymanthia Connell, M.D., LLC
Atlanta, Georgia USA

Second Edition: June 2020

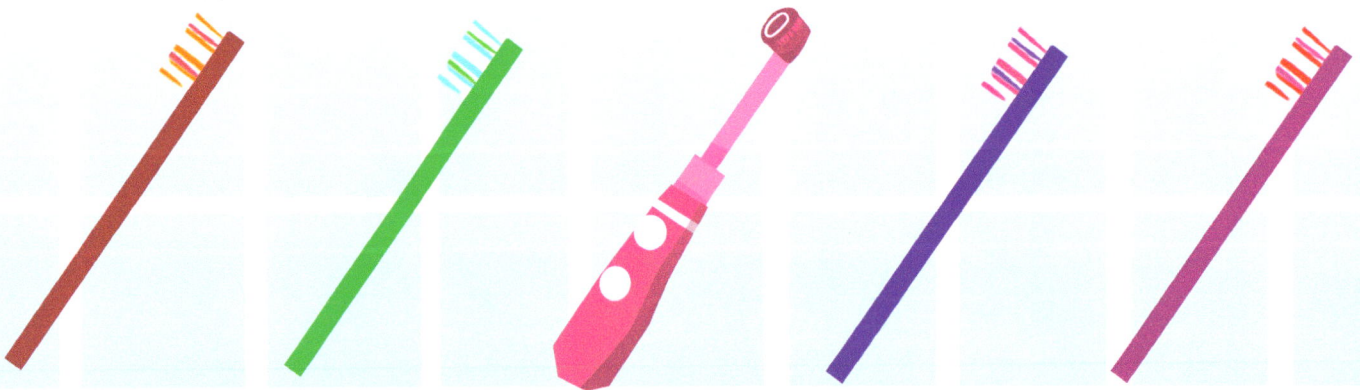

Samia
and Her
Electric
Toothbrush

By Dr. Cymanthia Connell
and Adam Ali

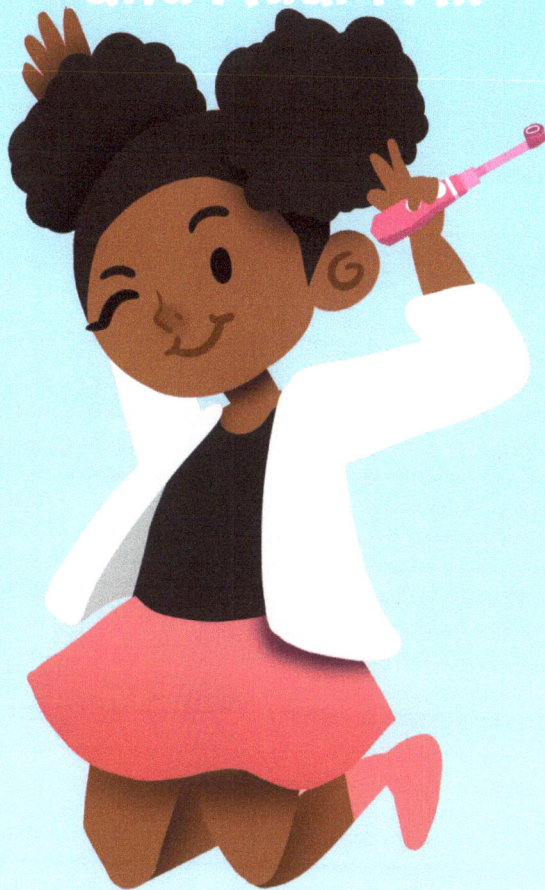

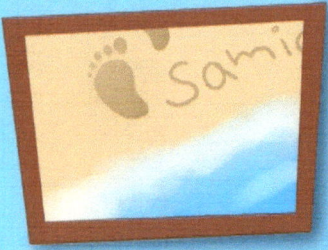

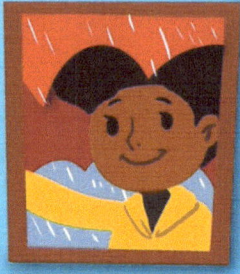

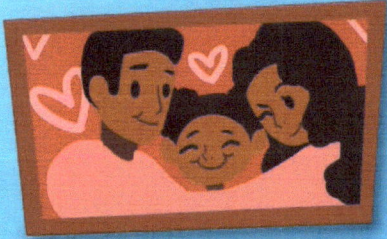

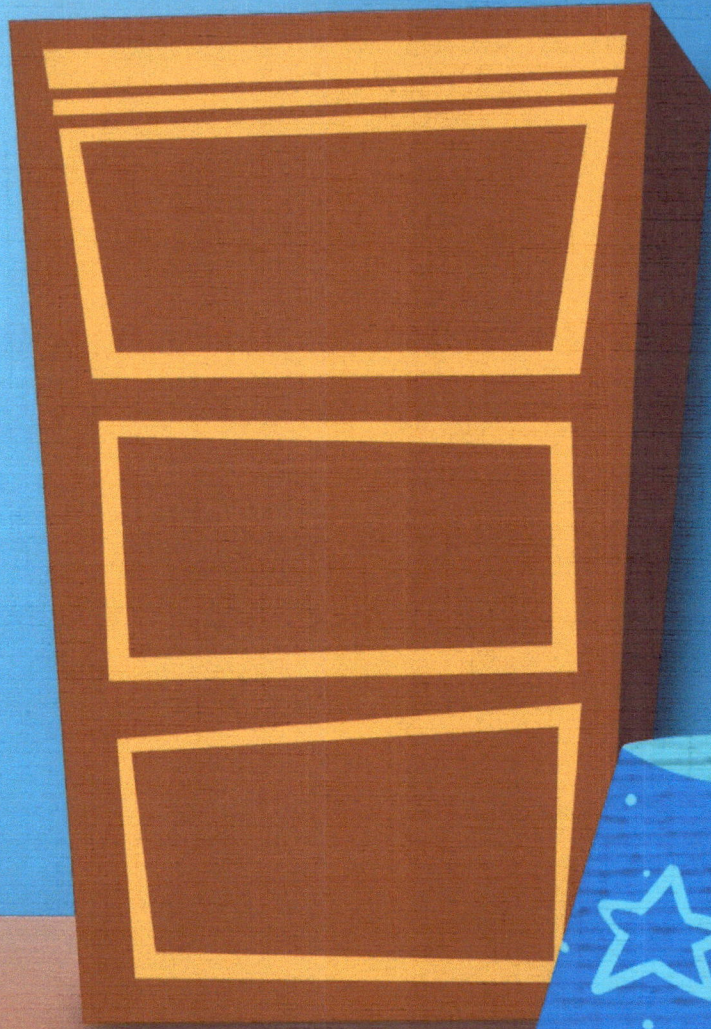

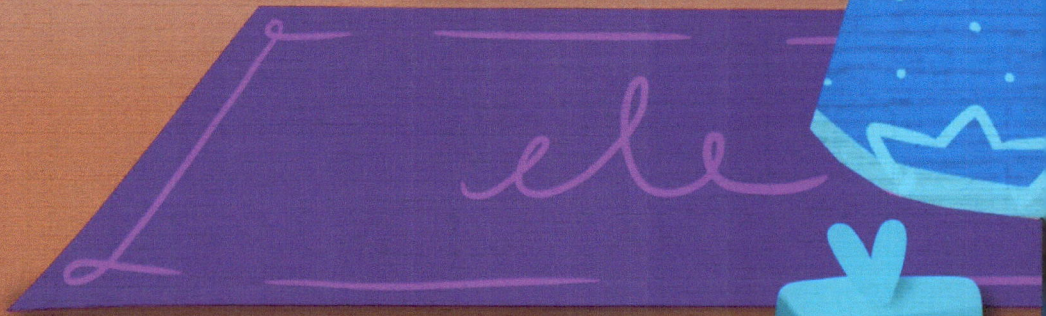

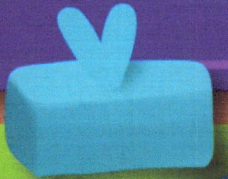

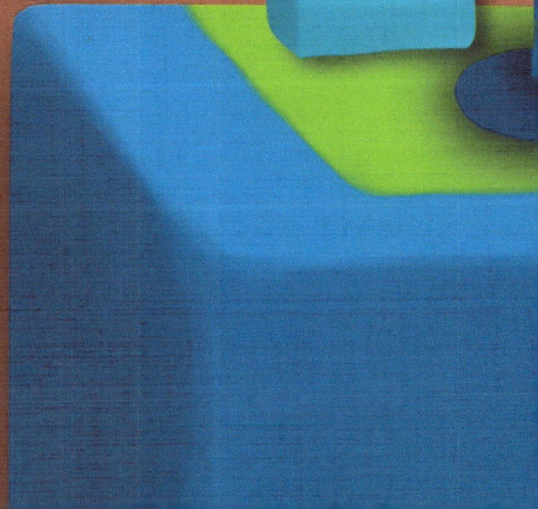

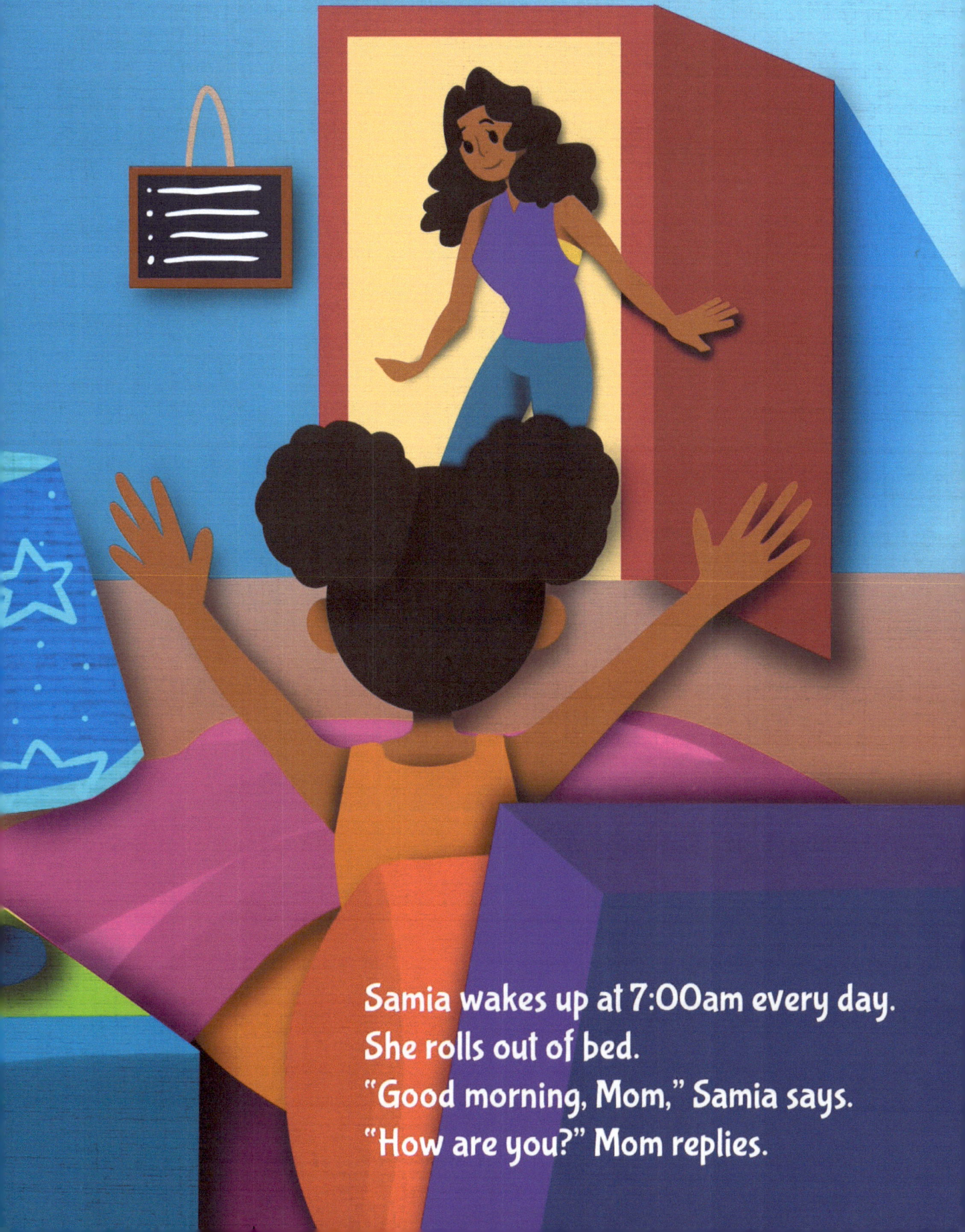

Samia wakes up at 7:00am every day.
She rolls out of bed.
"Good morning, Mom," Samia says.
"How are you?" Mom replies.

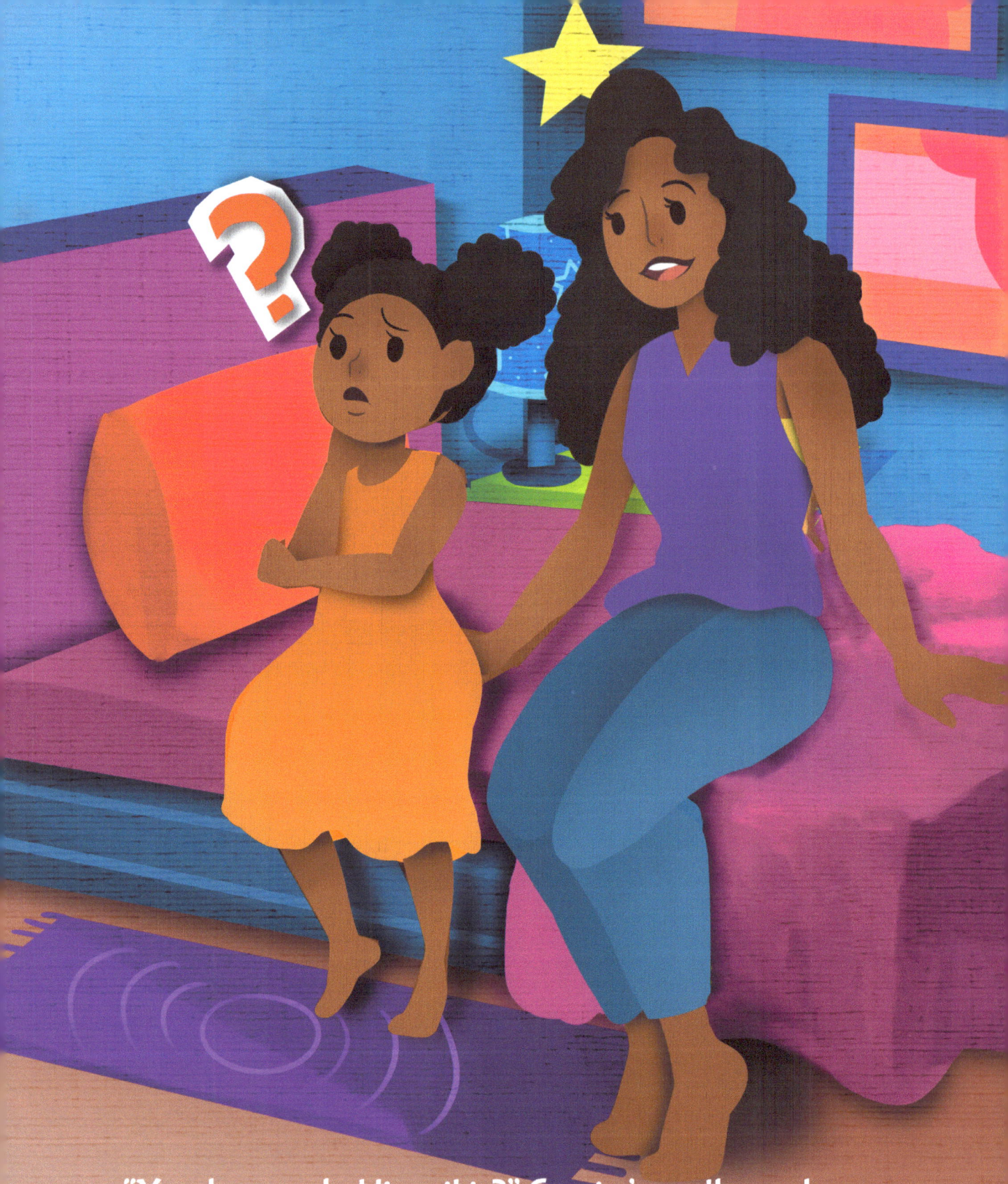

"You know what time it is?" Samia's mother asks.
Samia looks around, trying to remember what time it is.

"It's tooth–brushing time!"
Samia is happy.
"Yay!" Samia says and jumps up.

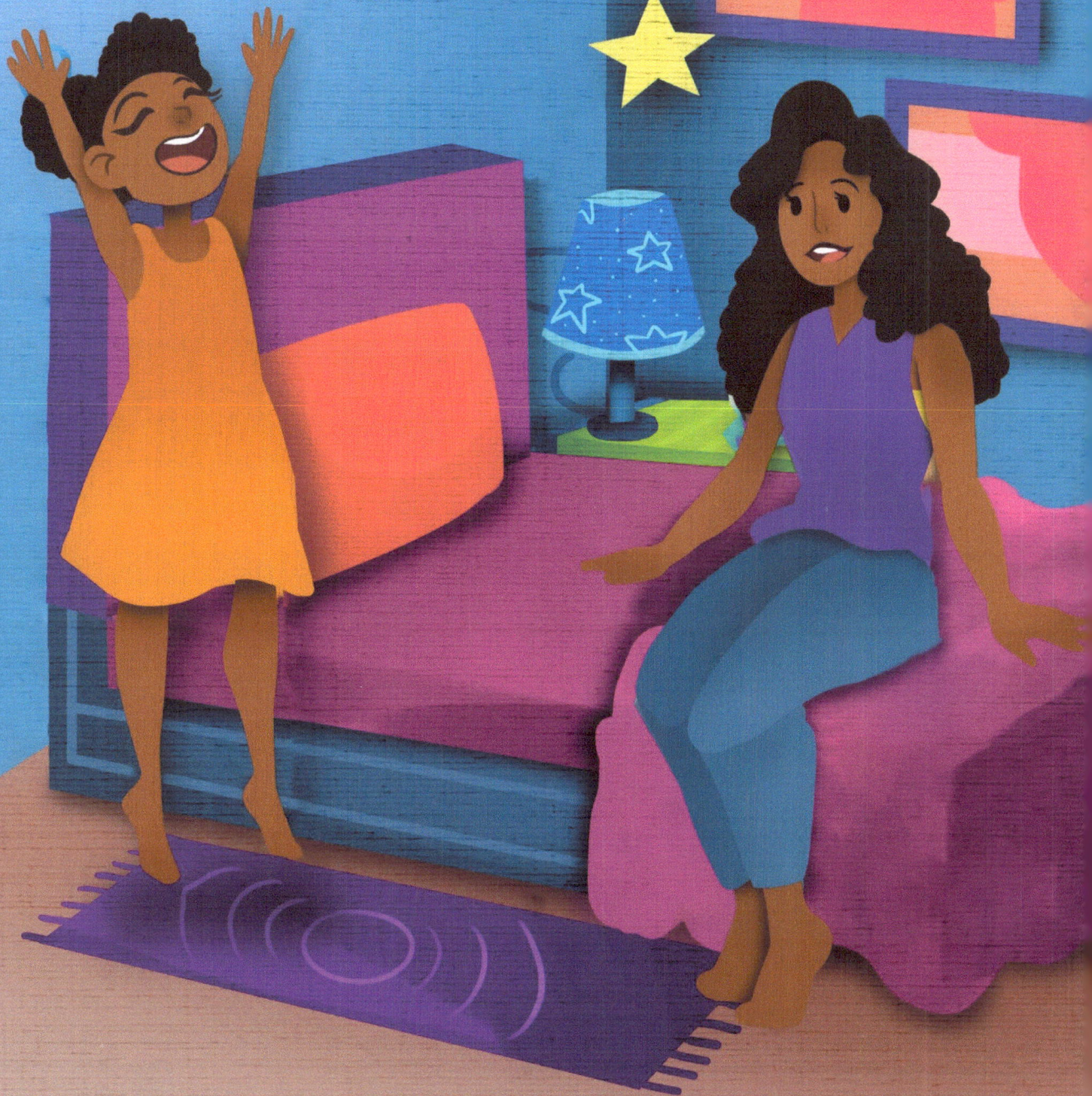

Samia gets to use her electric toothbrush again. Her father bought it as a gift for her birthday.

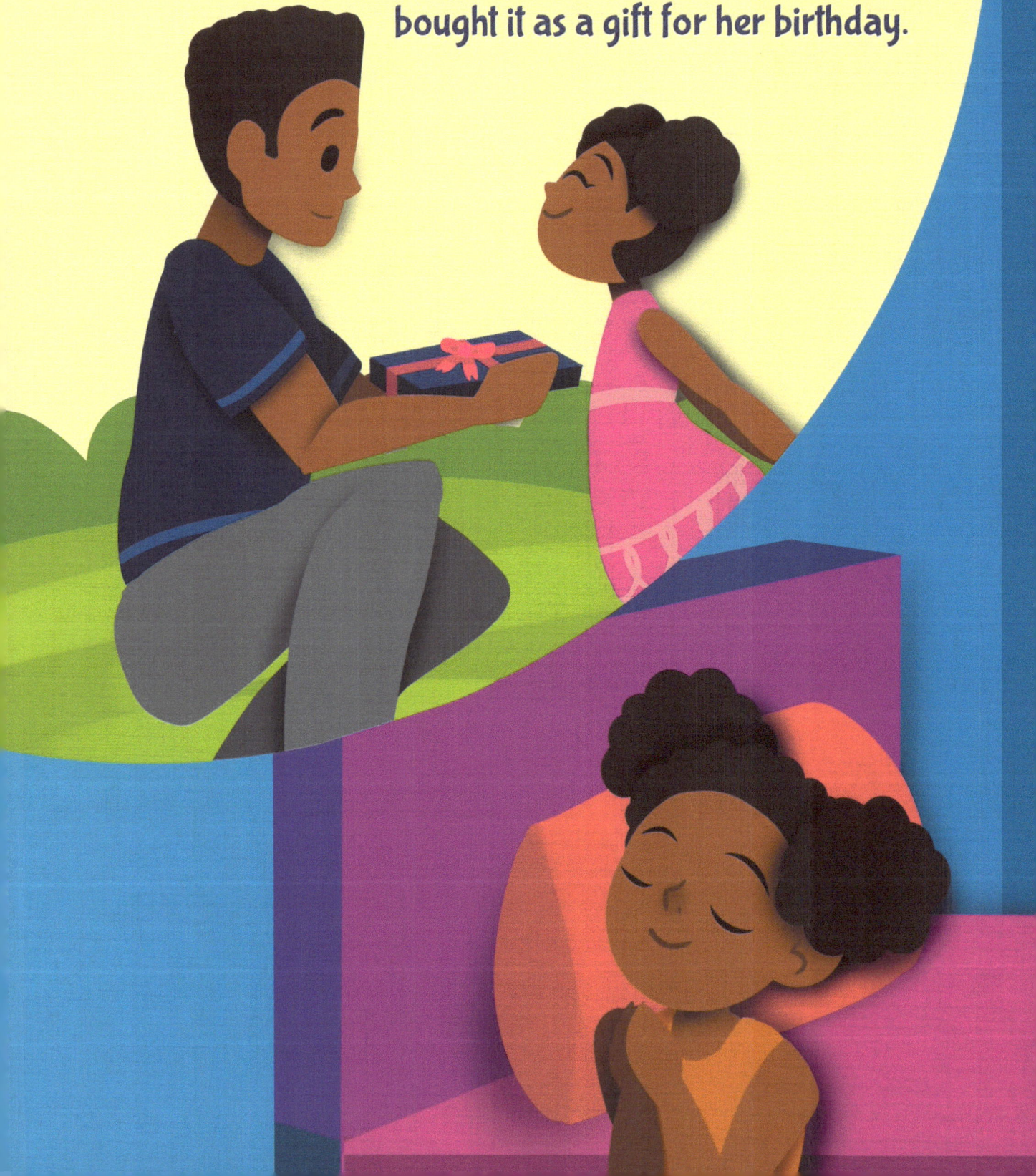

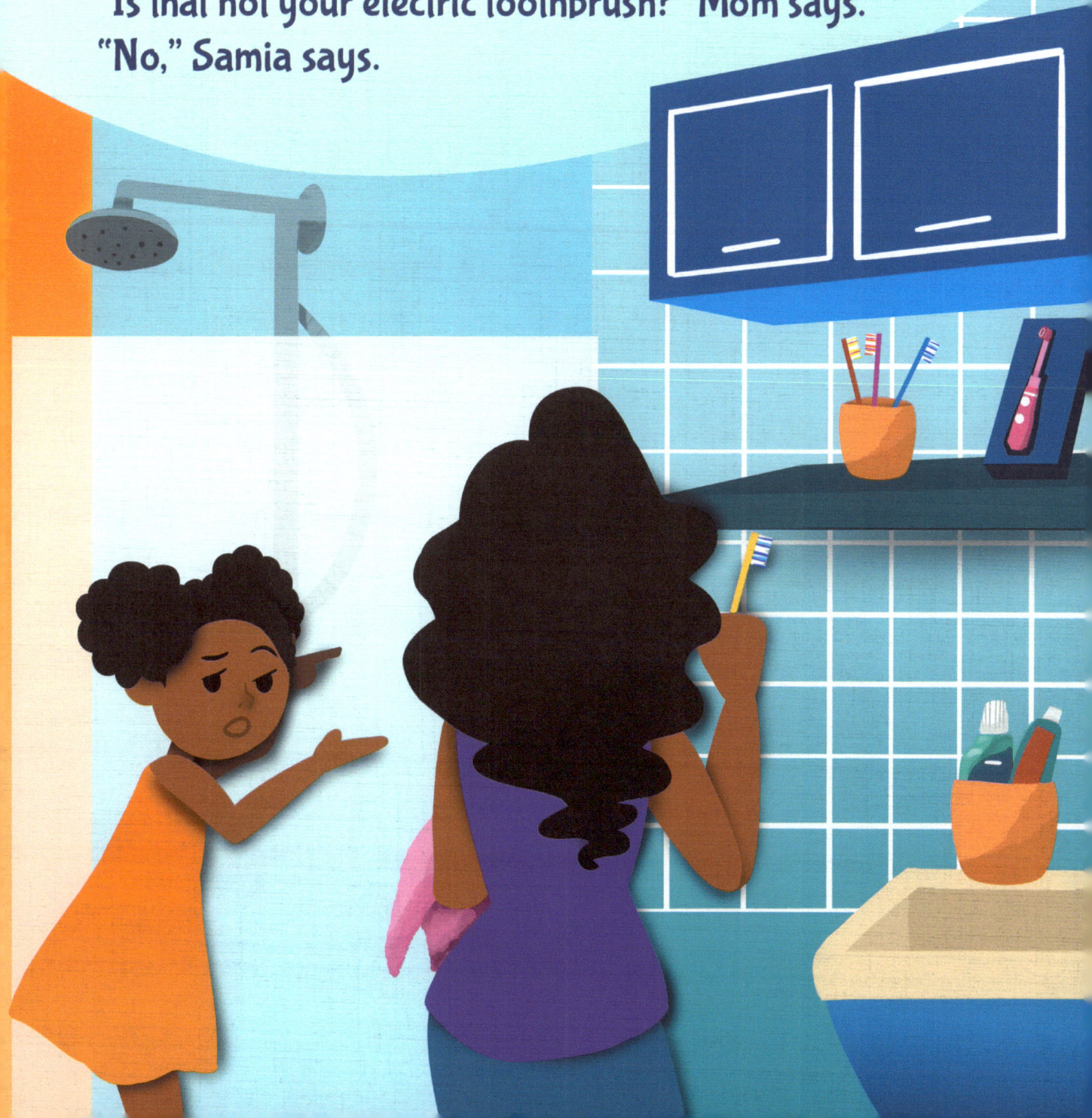

Mom gives her a toothbrush, but it's not her electric toothbrush.
"Mom, where is my toothbrush?" Samia asks.
Her mother smiles.
"Is that not your electric toothbrush?" Mom says.
"No," Samia says.

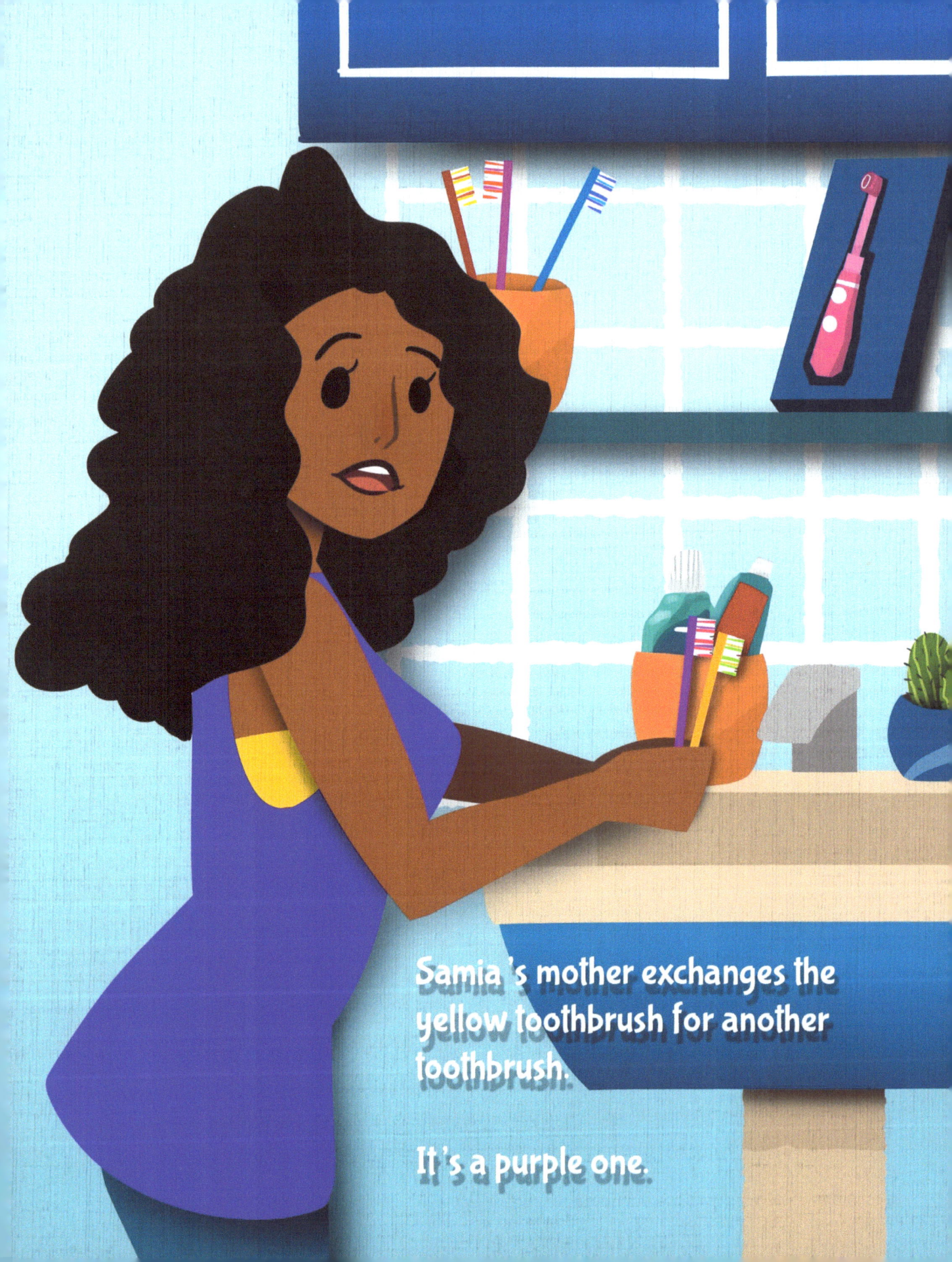

Samia's mother exchanges the yellow toothbrush for another toothbrush.

It's a purple one.

"But this is not my electric toothbrush either, Mom," Samia says.

"Oh! Sorry, Samia." Mom was teasing her on purpose!

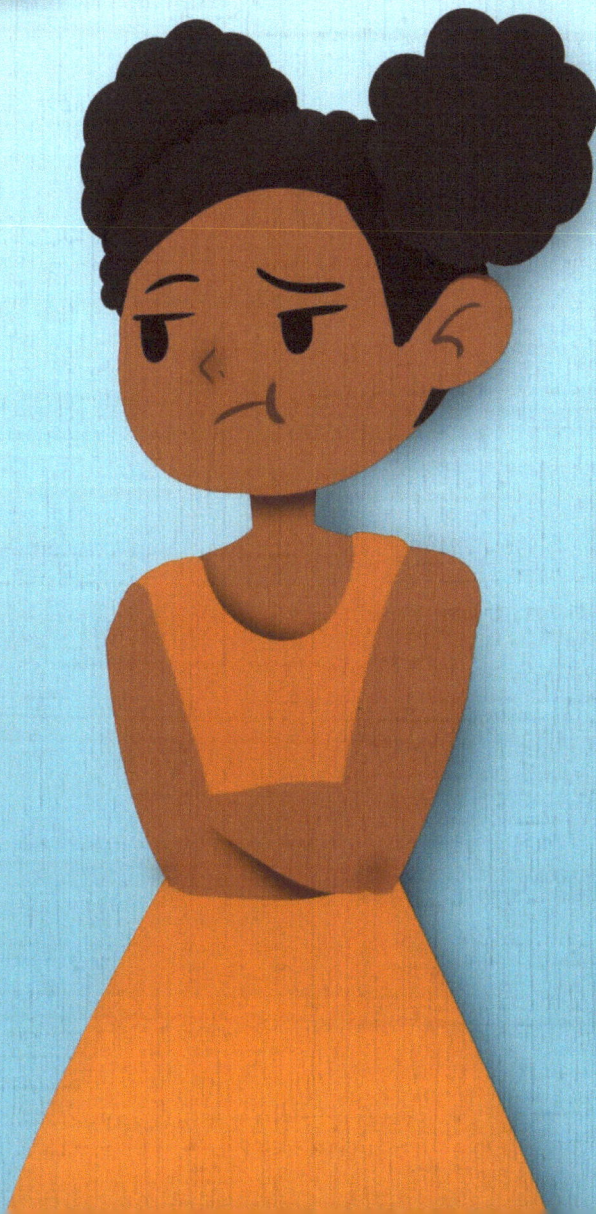

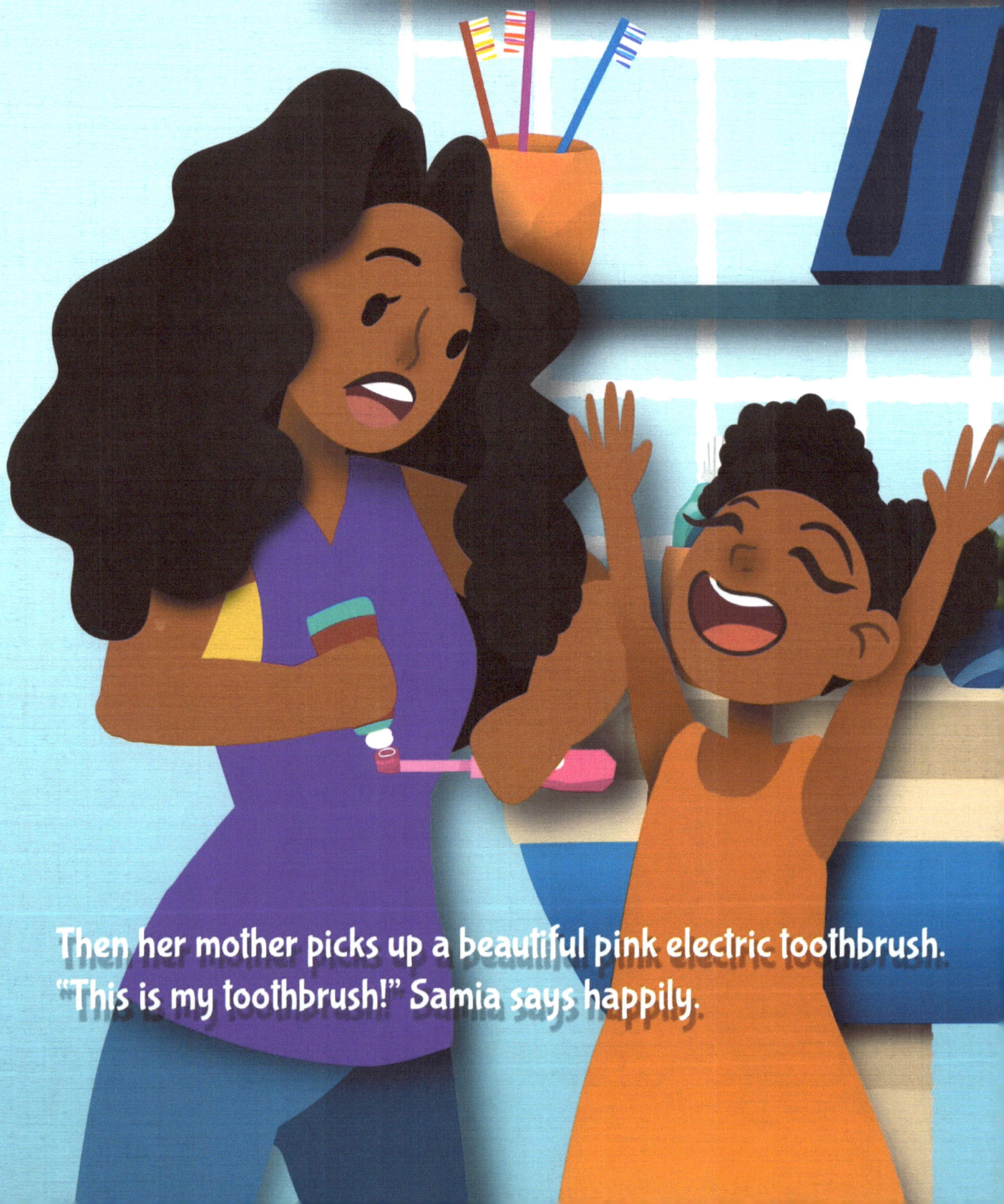

Then her mother picks up a beautiful pink electric toothbrush.
"This is my toothbrush!" Samia says happily.

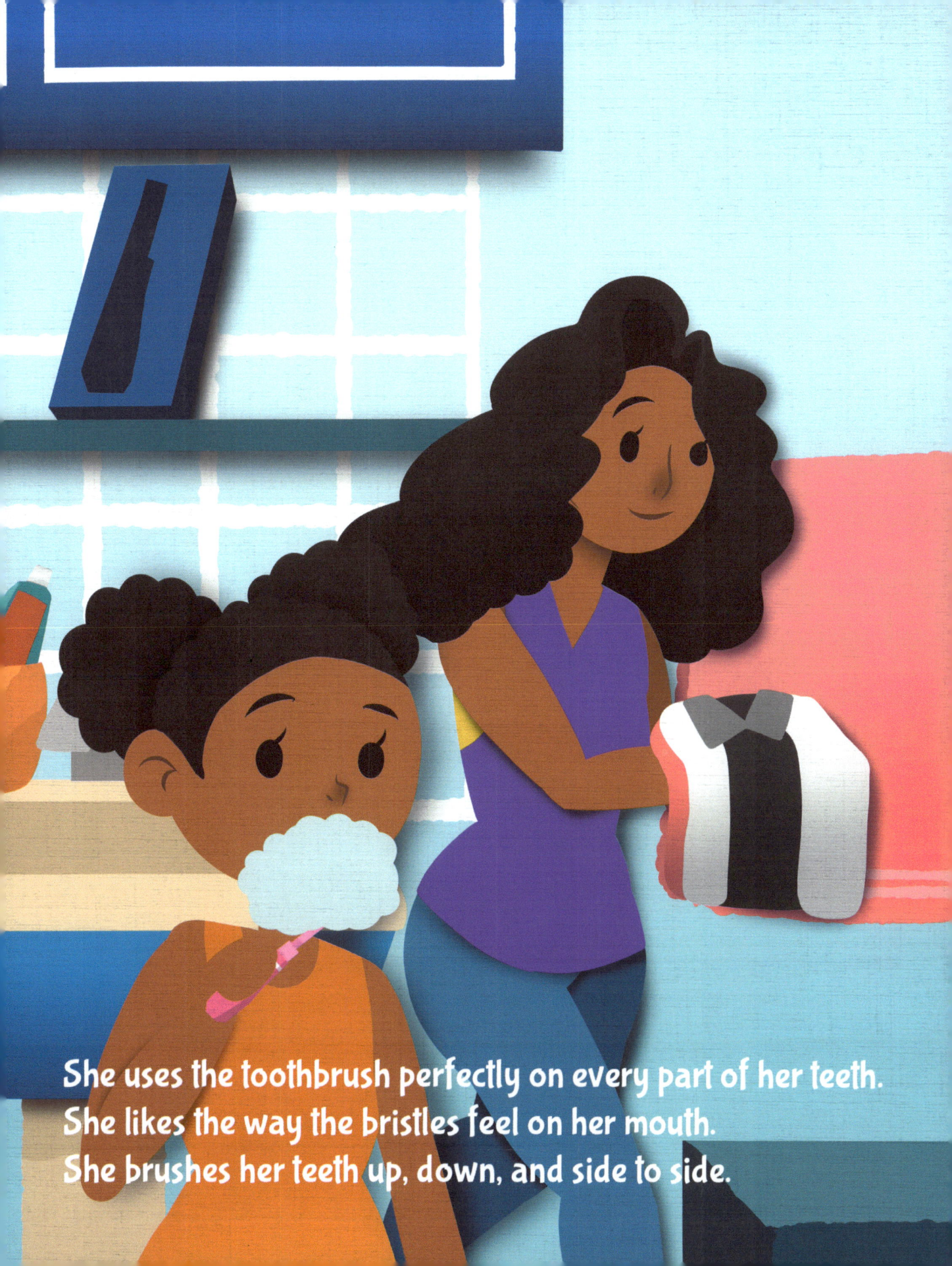

She uses the toothbrush perfectly on every part of her teeth.
She likes the way the bristles feel on her mouth.
She brushes her teeth up, down, and side to side.

"Oh dear, Samia, you'll be late for school," Mom says.

Samia stops and looks sadly at her toothbrush.

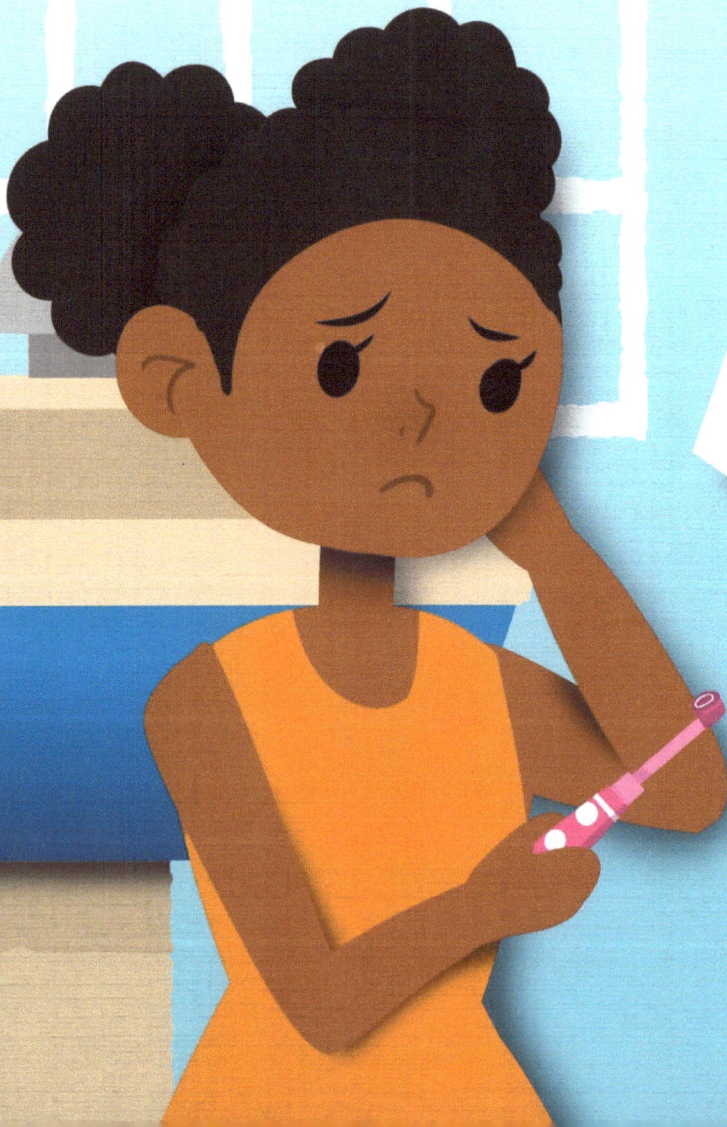

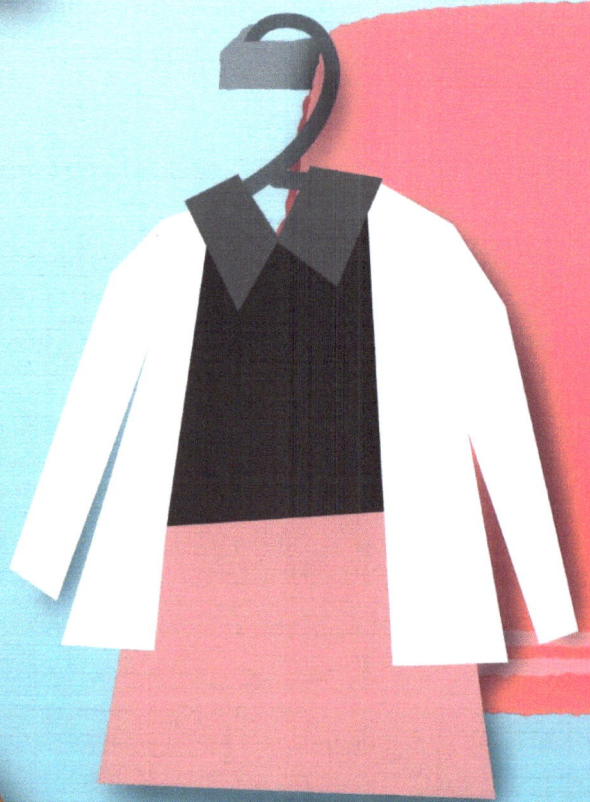

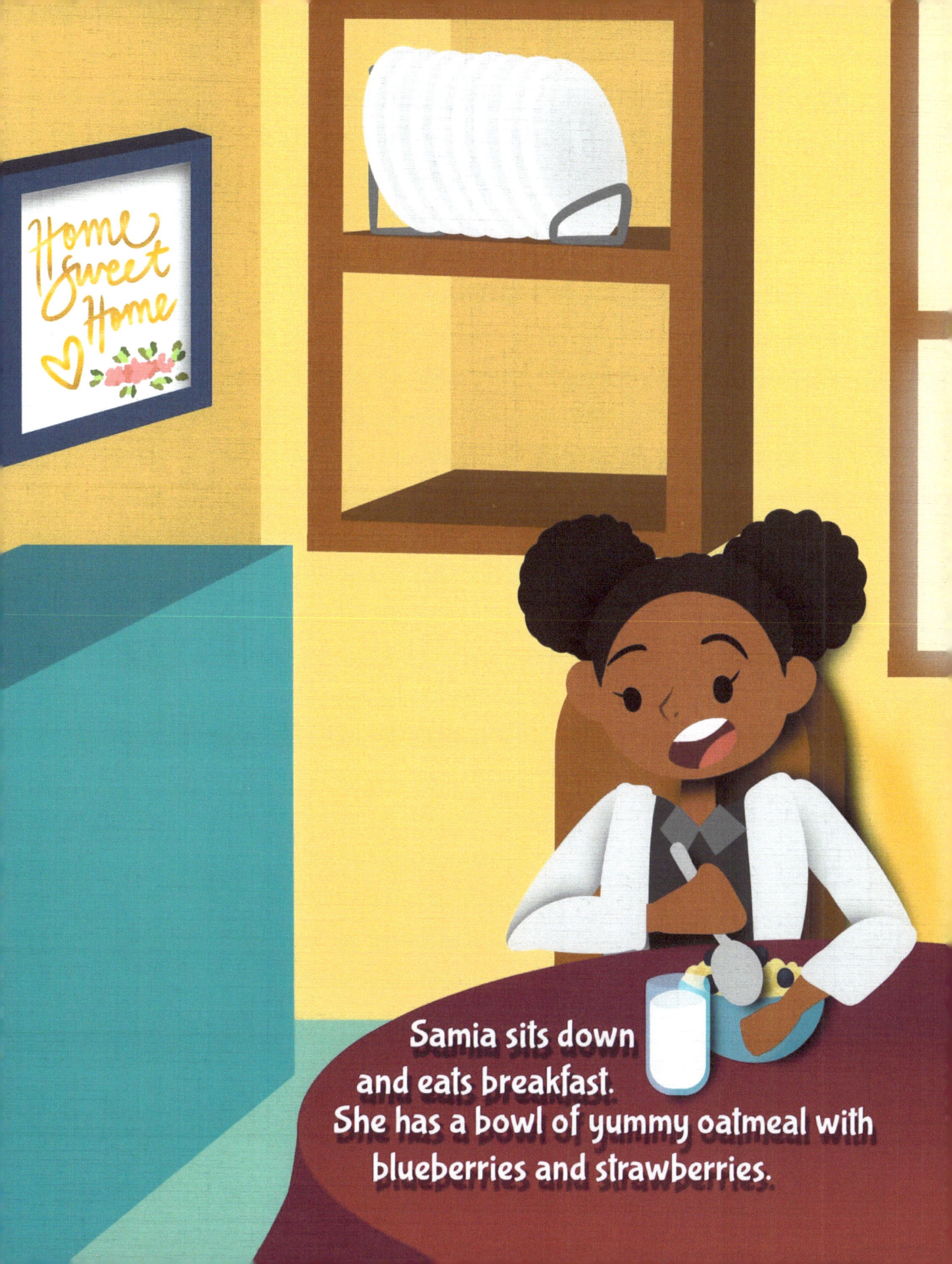

Samia sits down
and eats breakfast.
She has a bowl of yummy oatmeal with
blueberries and strawberries.

After breakfast, Samia rushes to the bathroom.
Samia's mother follows her.

Samia loves the electric toothbrush.
She tries to reach for it on the shelf,
but it was a bit too high for her.

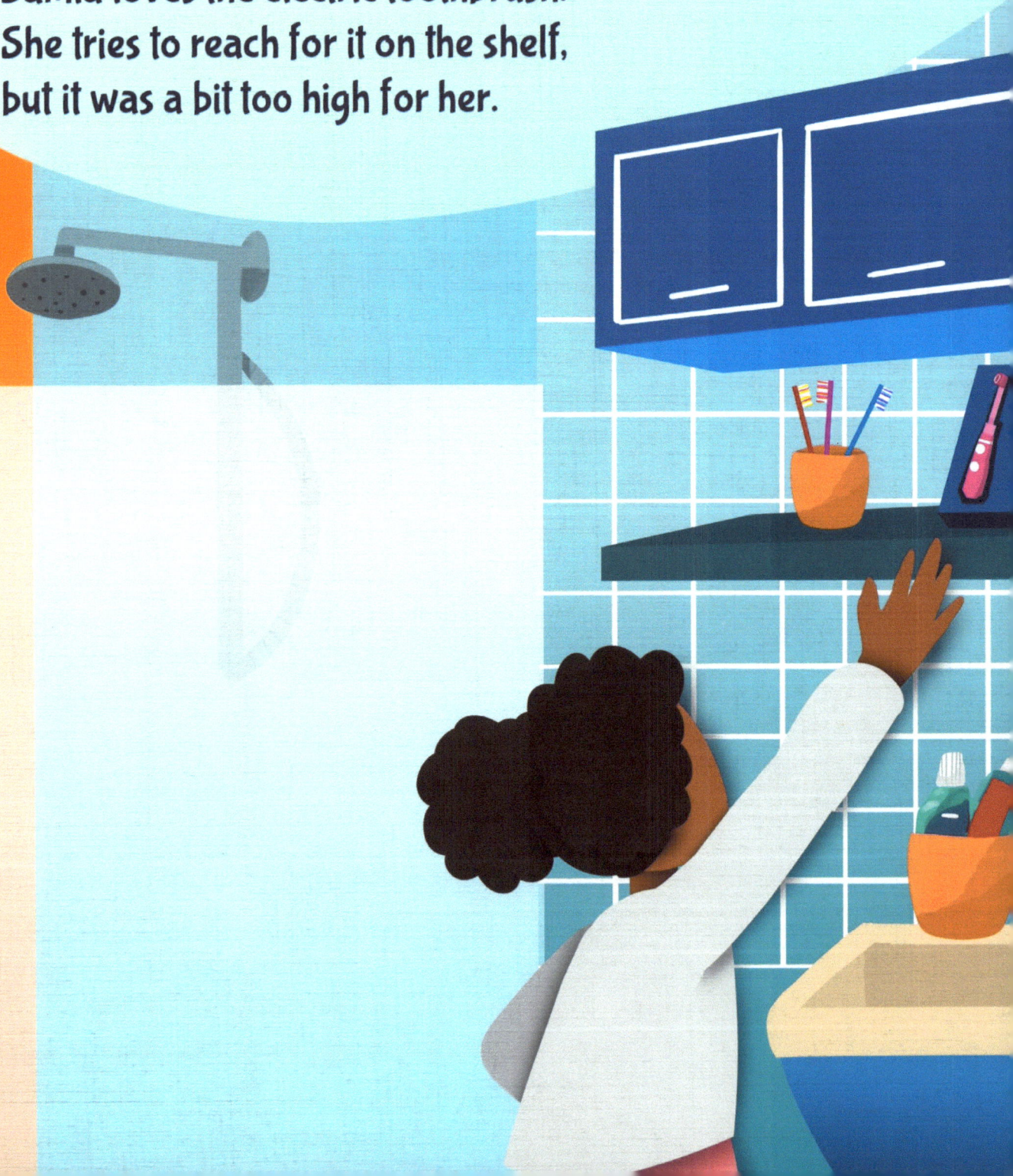

"Samia, can I help you get your electric toothbrush?" Mom asks.

"Yes, please," Samia says.

Samia brushes her teeth one last time before heading to school.

"And I will show it to my friends for show—and—tell."

"That will be great!" Mom says.

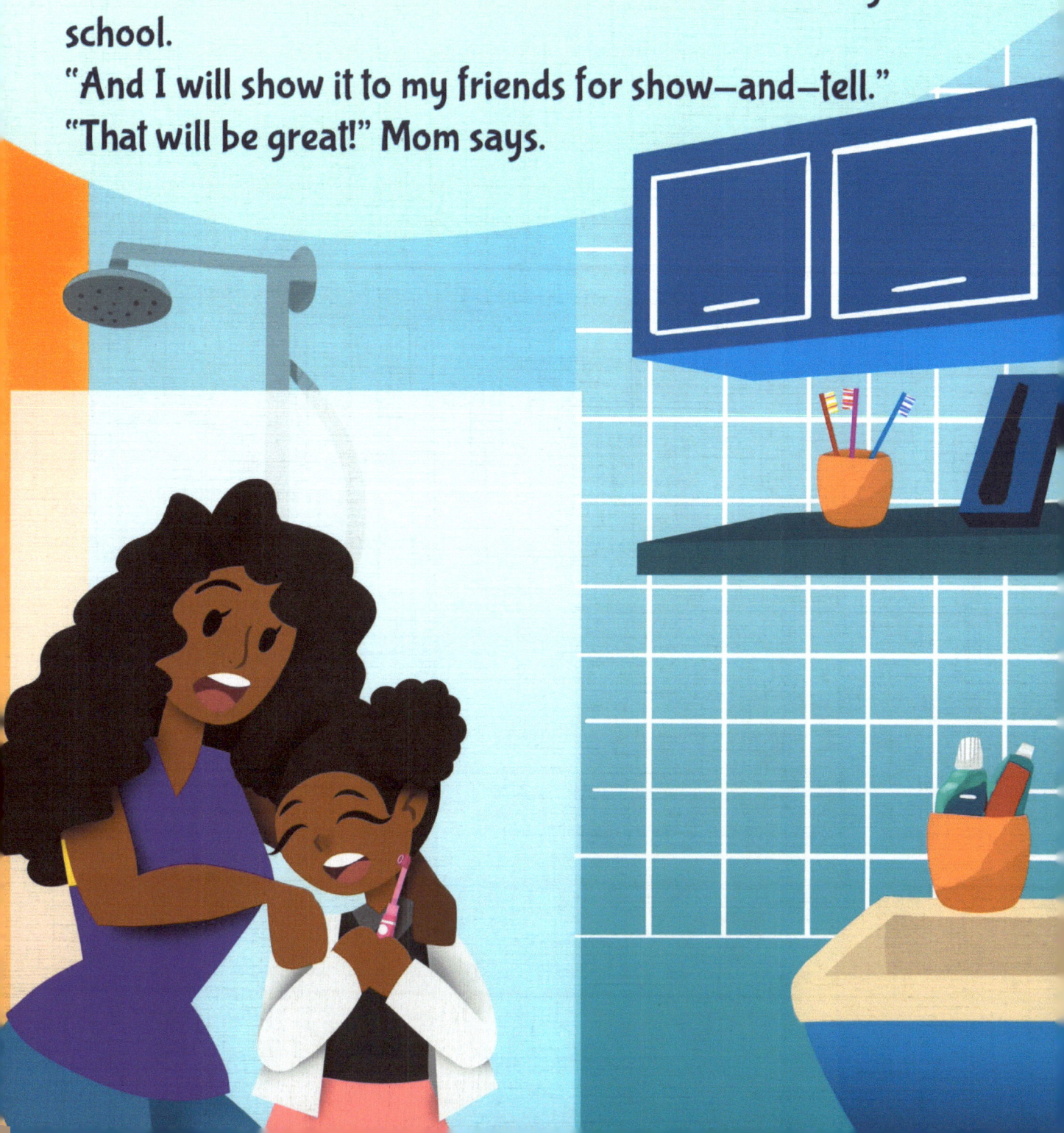

During show—and—tell, Samia stands tall and says, "This is my toothbrush. It's the best toothbrush in the whole wide world!" Samia's toothbrush has a special button that makes the bristles spin around really fast. "When the bristles spin, they clean my teeth really well."

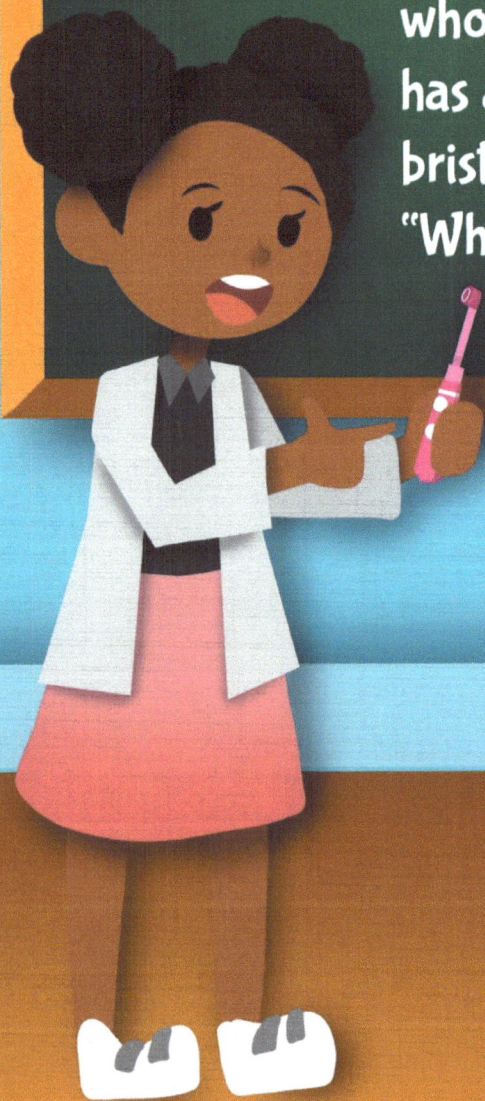

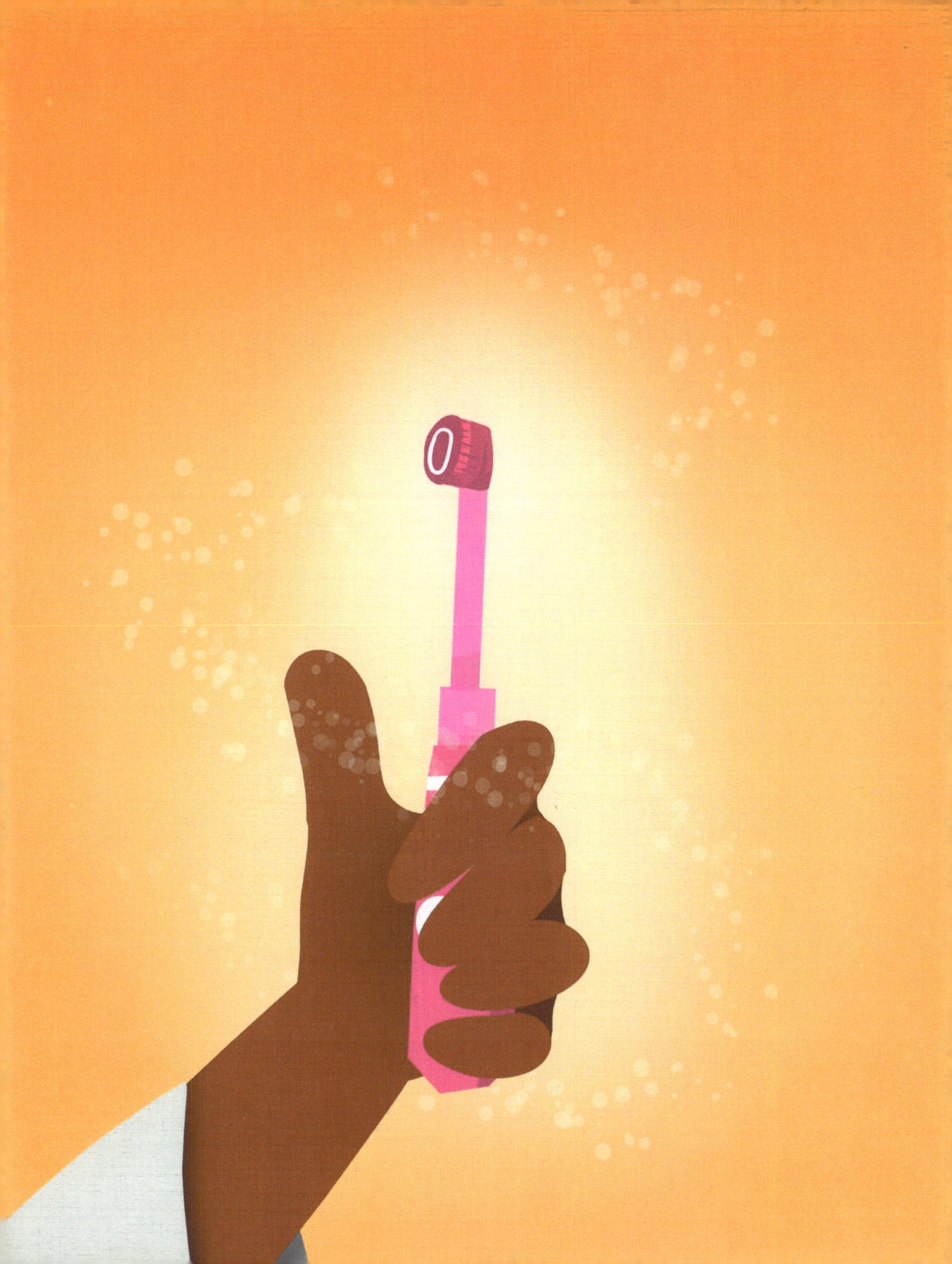

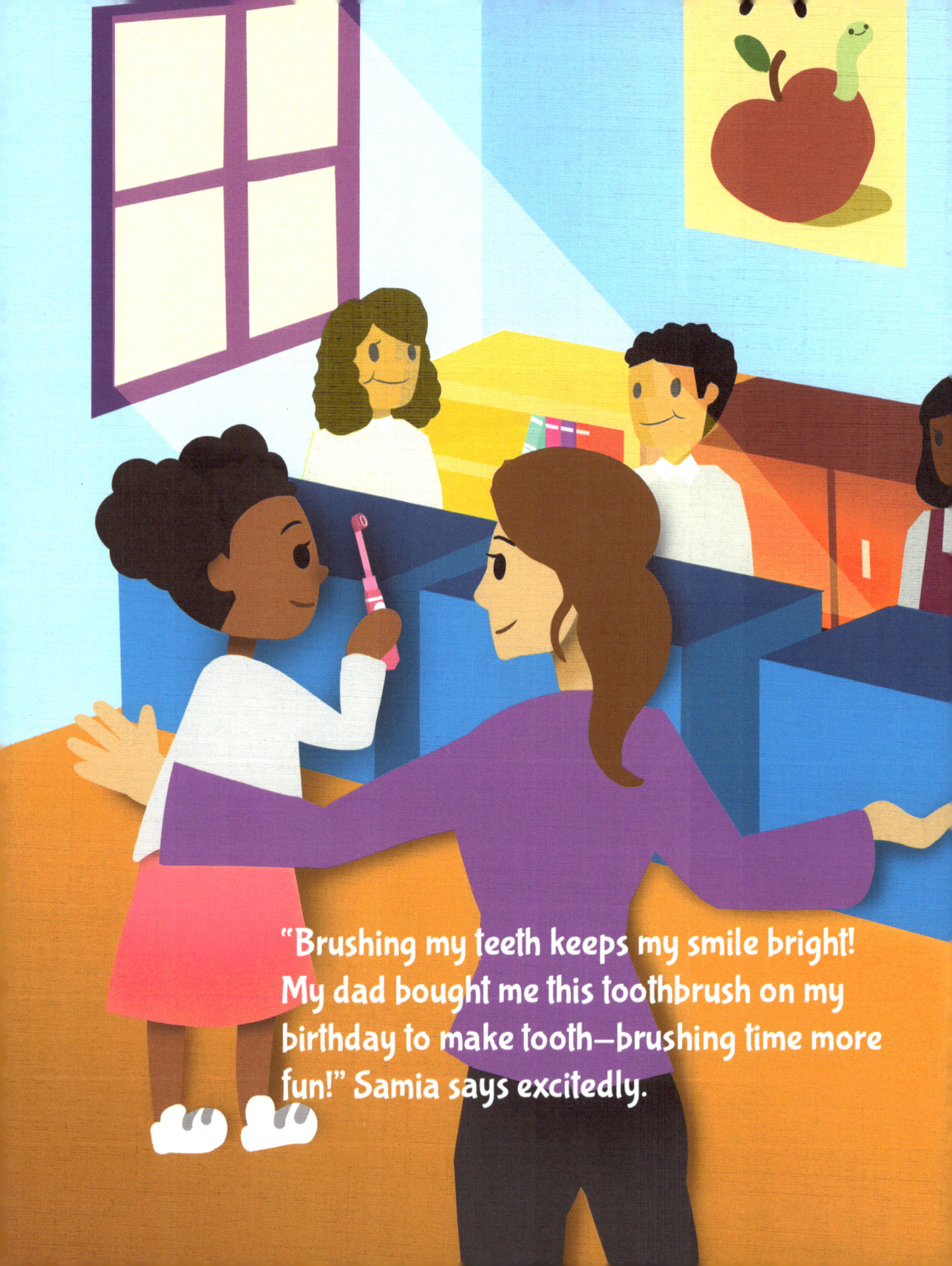

"Brushing my teeth keeps my smile bright! My dad bought me this toothbrush on my birthday to make tooth-brushing time more fun!" Samia says excitedly.

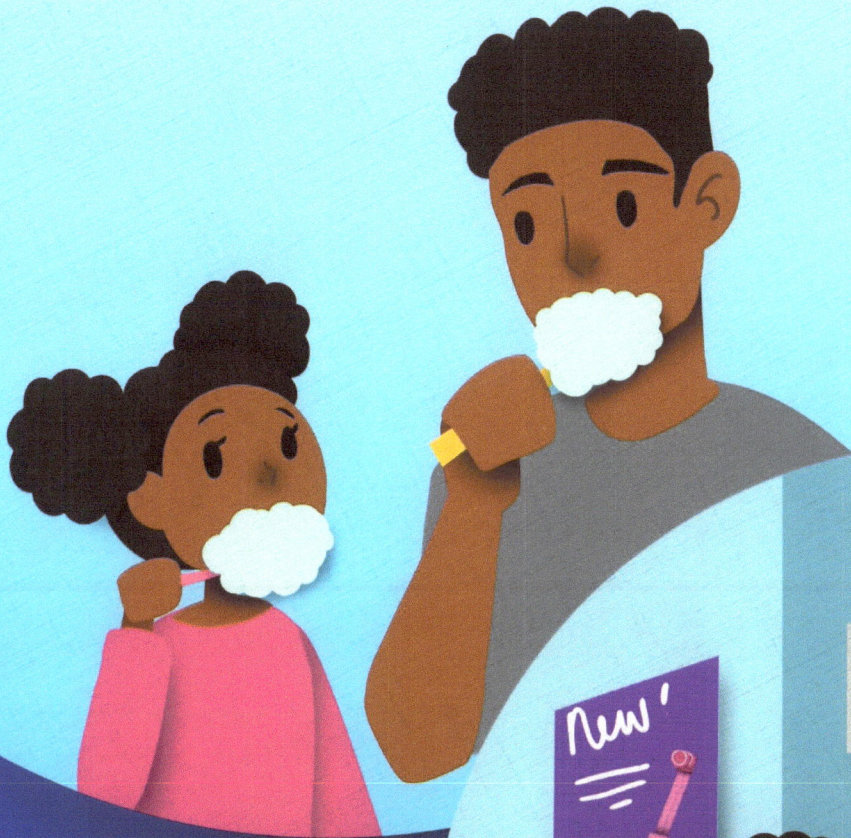

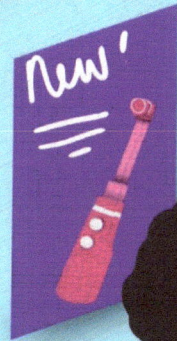

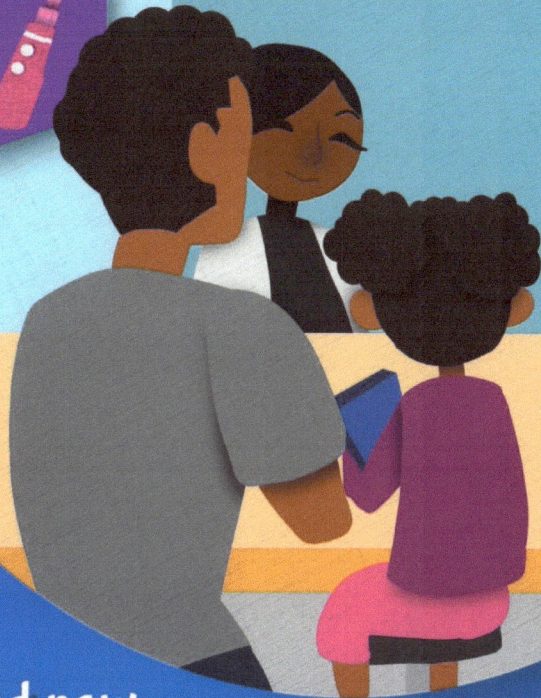

"My dad loves gadgets, and now
I have a special gadget too!"

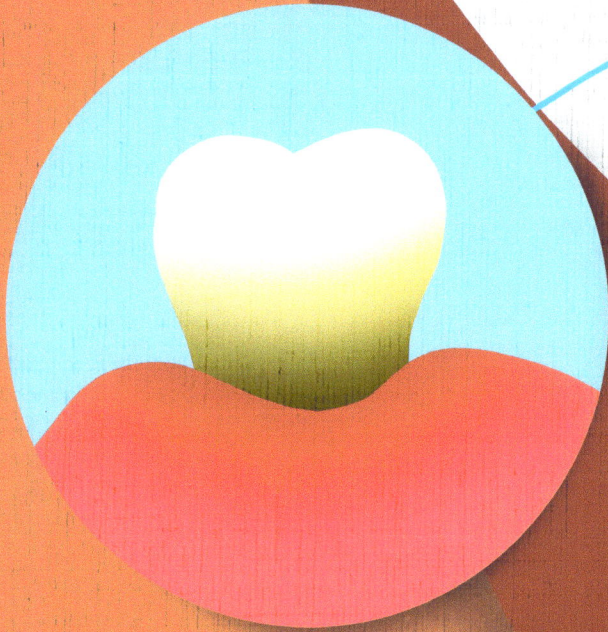

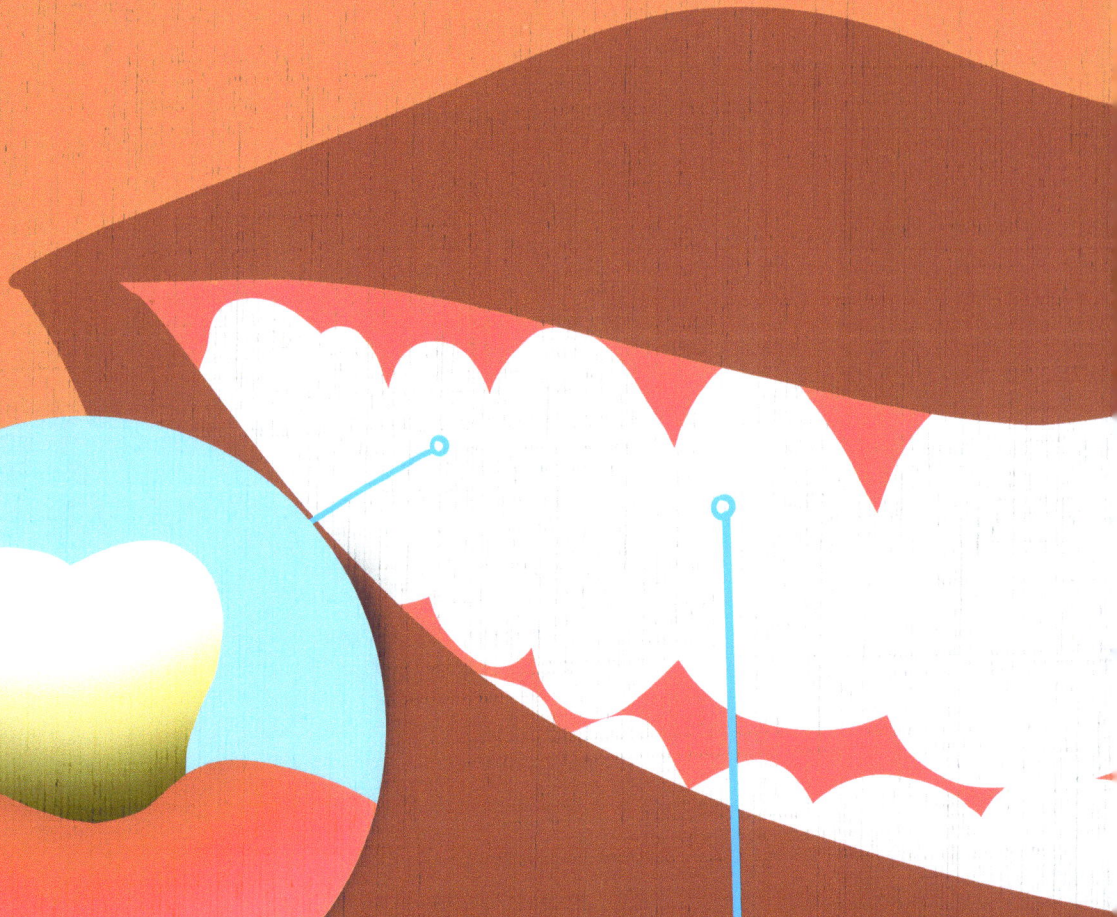

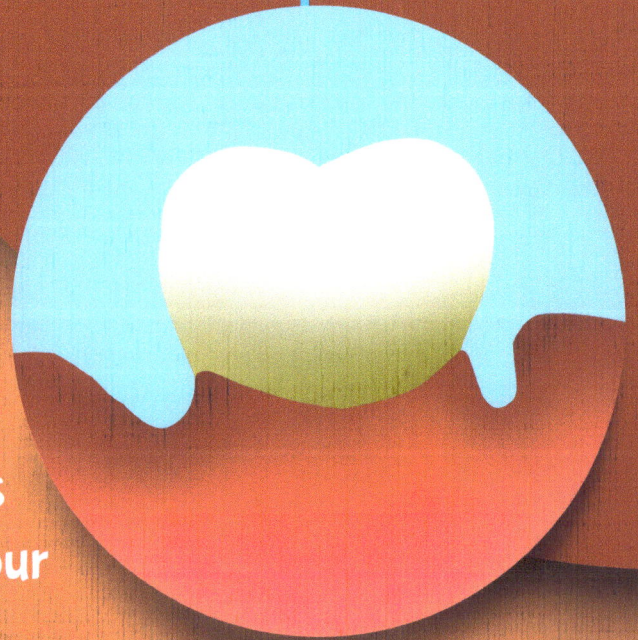

"Brushing your teeth is also important so you don't get plaque on your teeth. Plaque is from bad germs that stick to your teeth. And if you don't brush about twice a day, you can get gingivitis." Samia says.

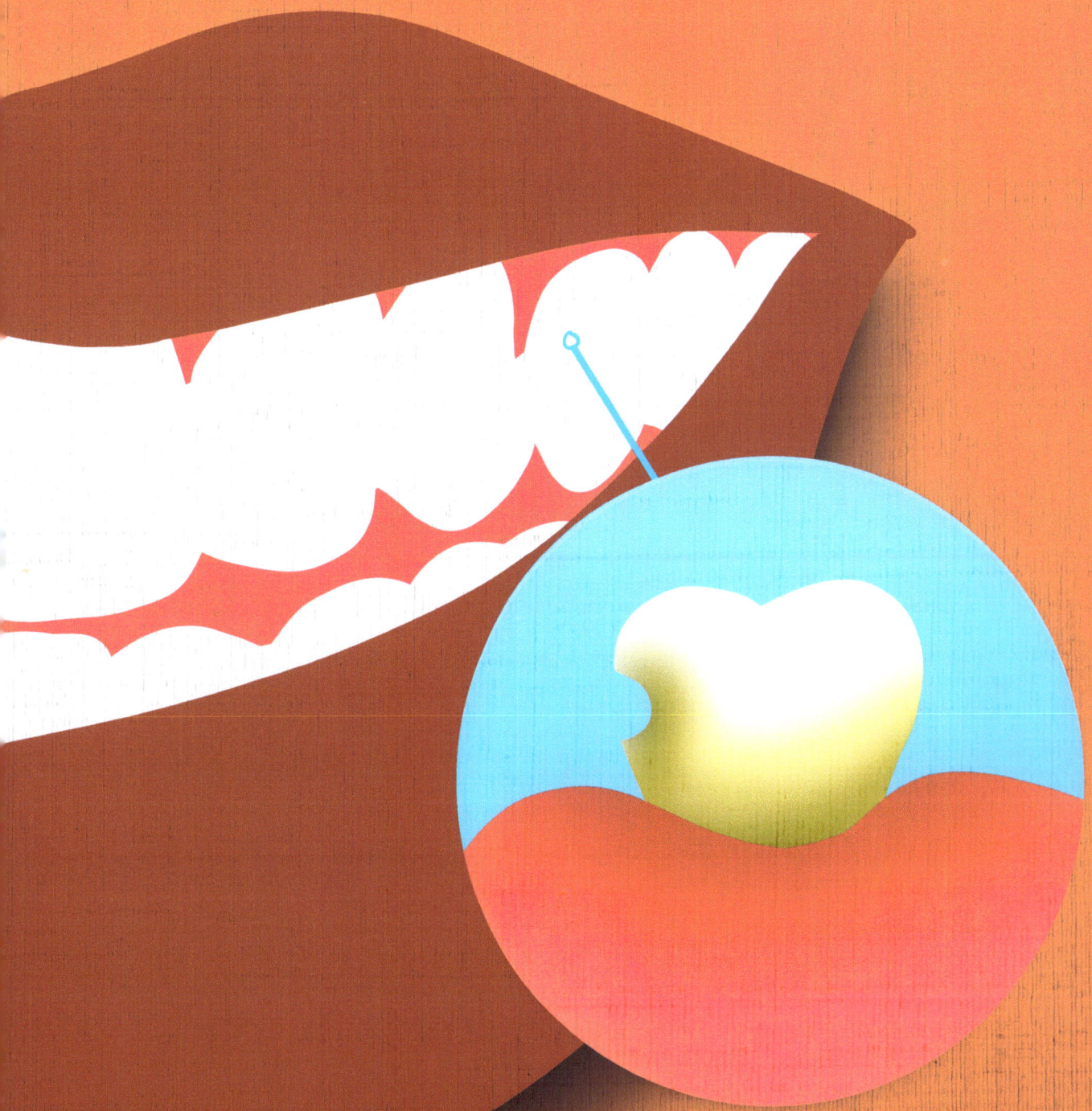

"Another reason you brush your teeth is so you don't get cavities. Cavities can really hurt your teeth."

During recess, Samia's best friend, Rupee, asks to look at her electric toothbrush again.
Samia is happy to show it to her.

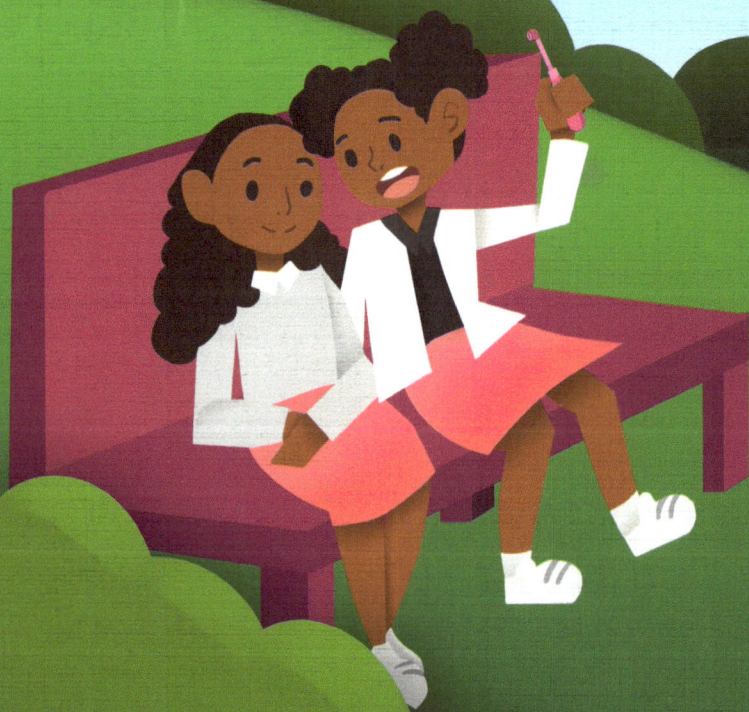

Samia shows Rupee what the button on her toothbrush can do.
"Wow! I think I 'll ask my dad for an electric toothbrush for my birthday," says Rupee.

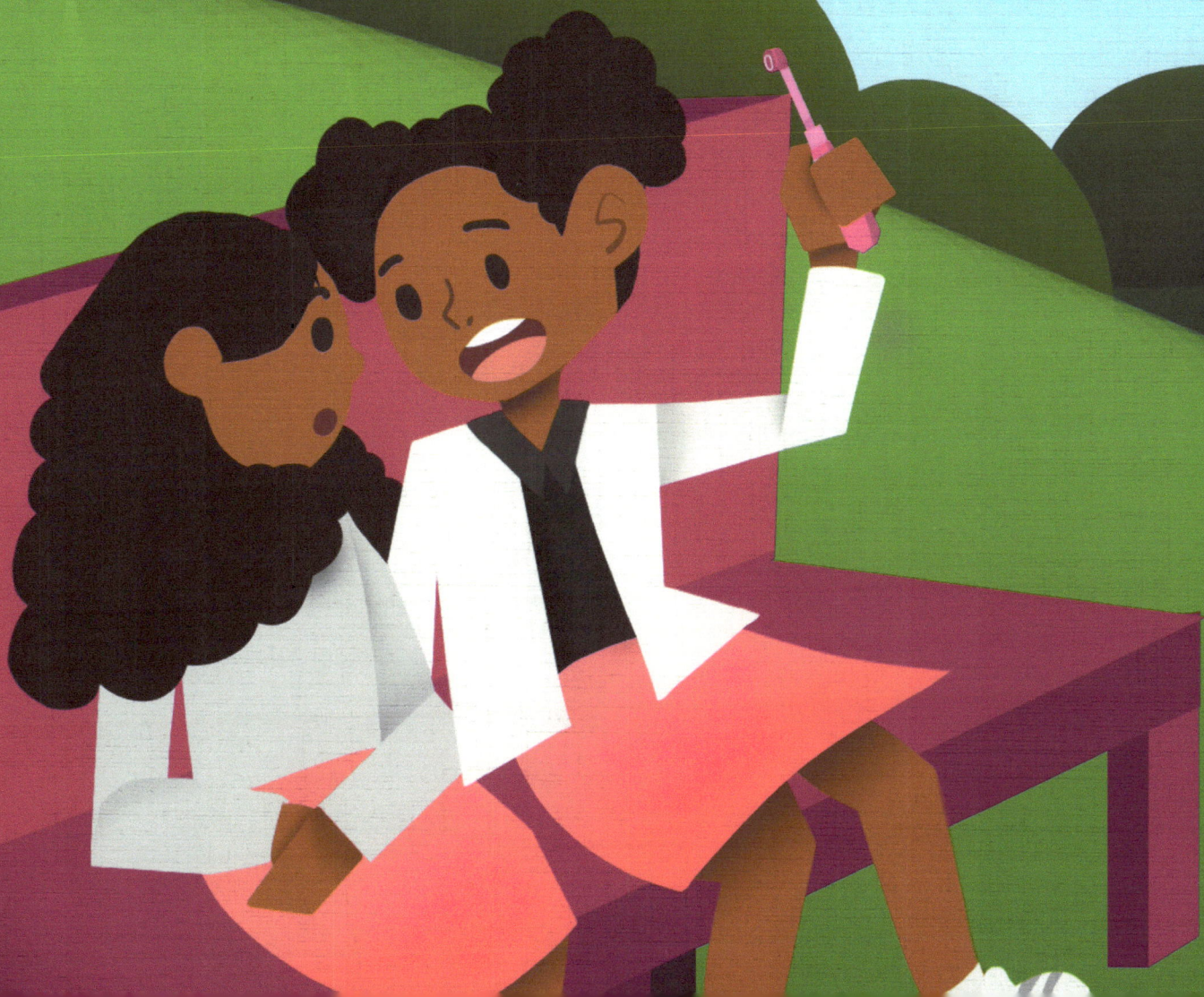

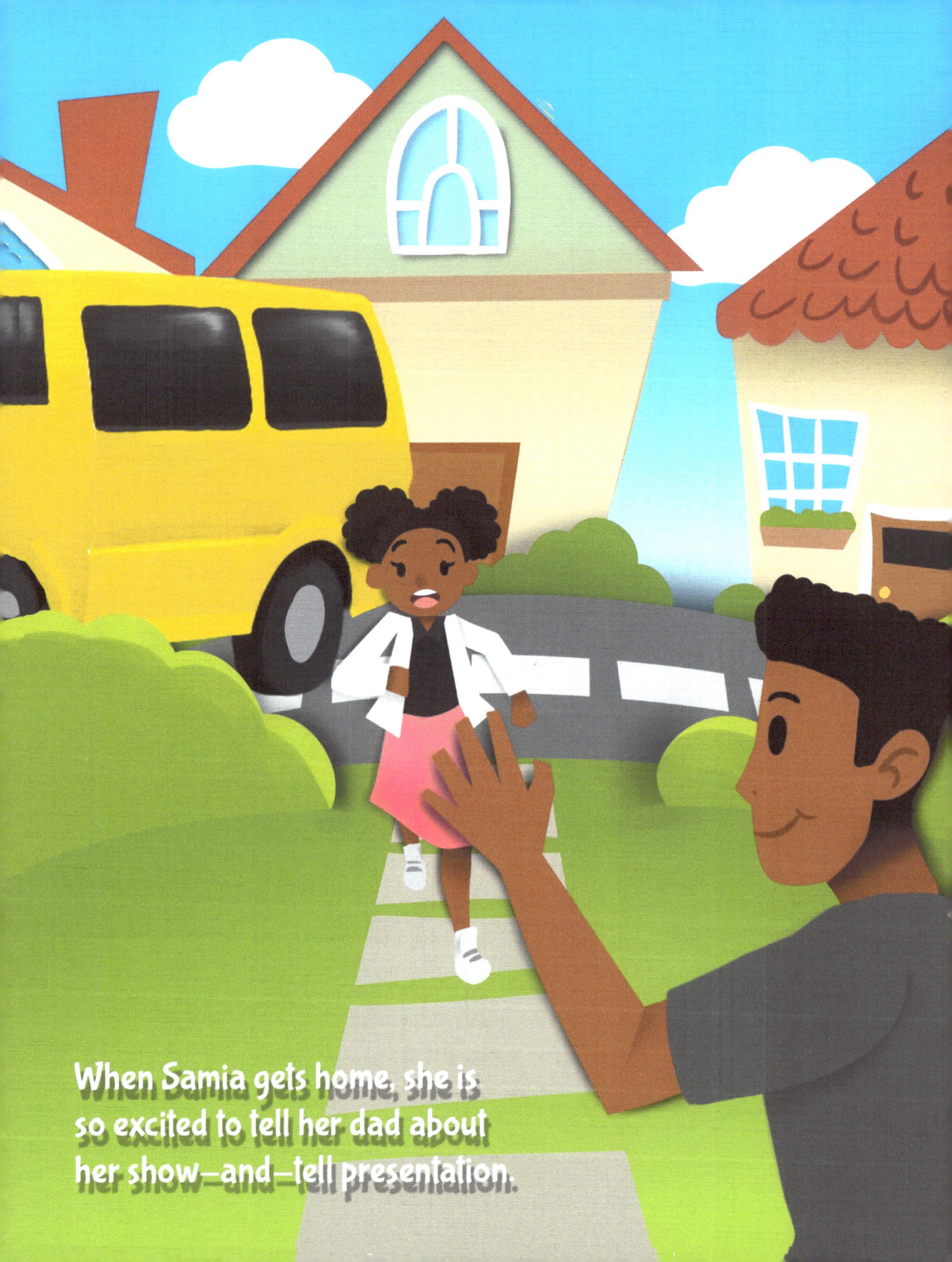

When Samia gets home, she is so excited to tell her dad about her show-and-tell presentation.

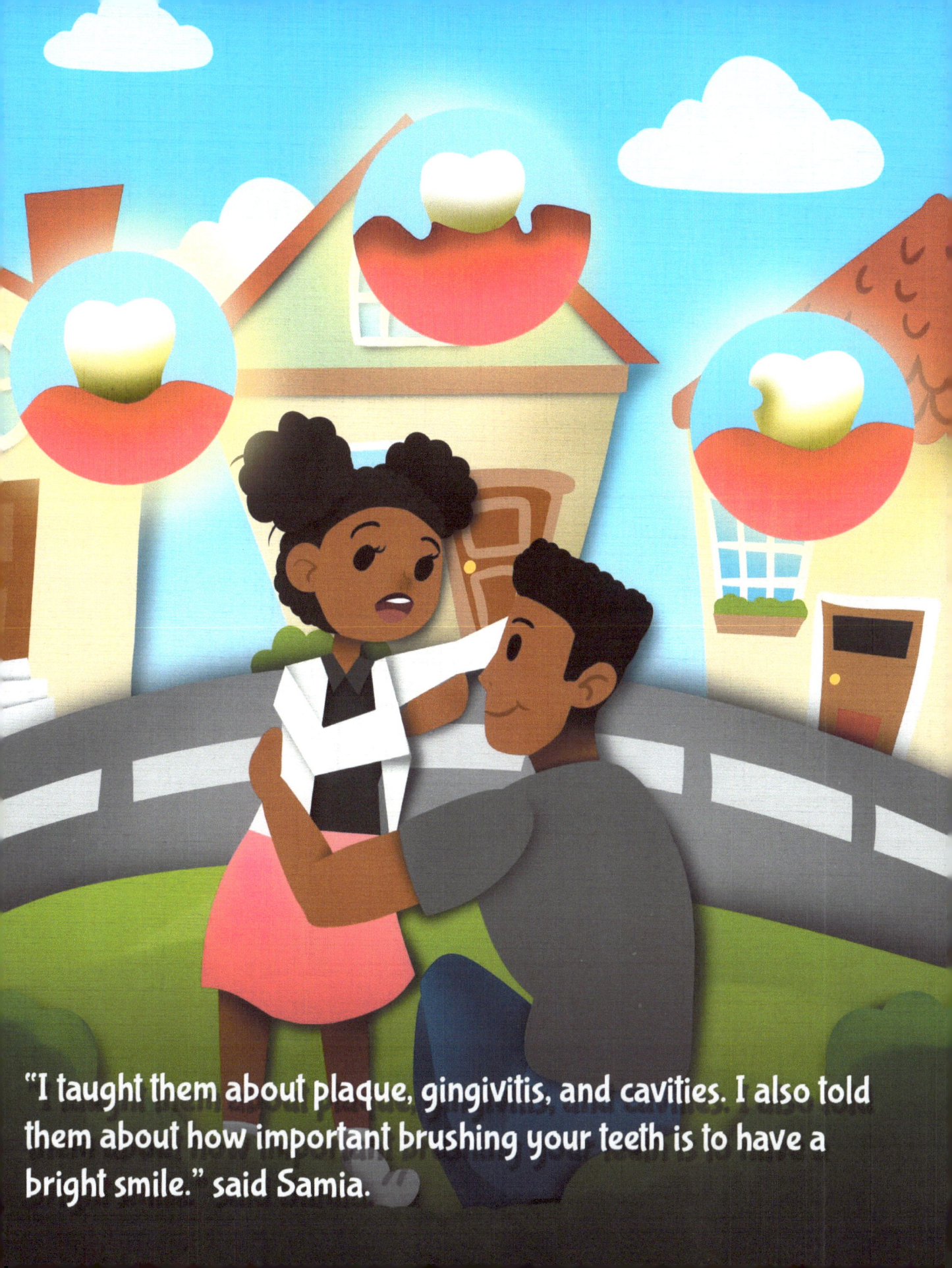

"I taught them about plaque, gingivitis, and cavities. I also told them about how important brushing your teeth is to have a bright smile." said Samia.

"I'm so proud of you," Samia's dad says as he gives her a big hug.
"I'm proud of me too," Samia says with a smile.

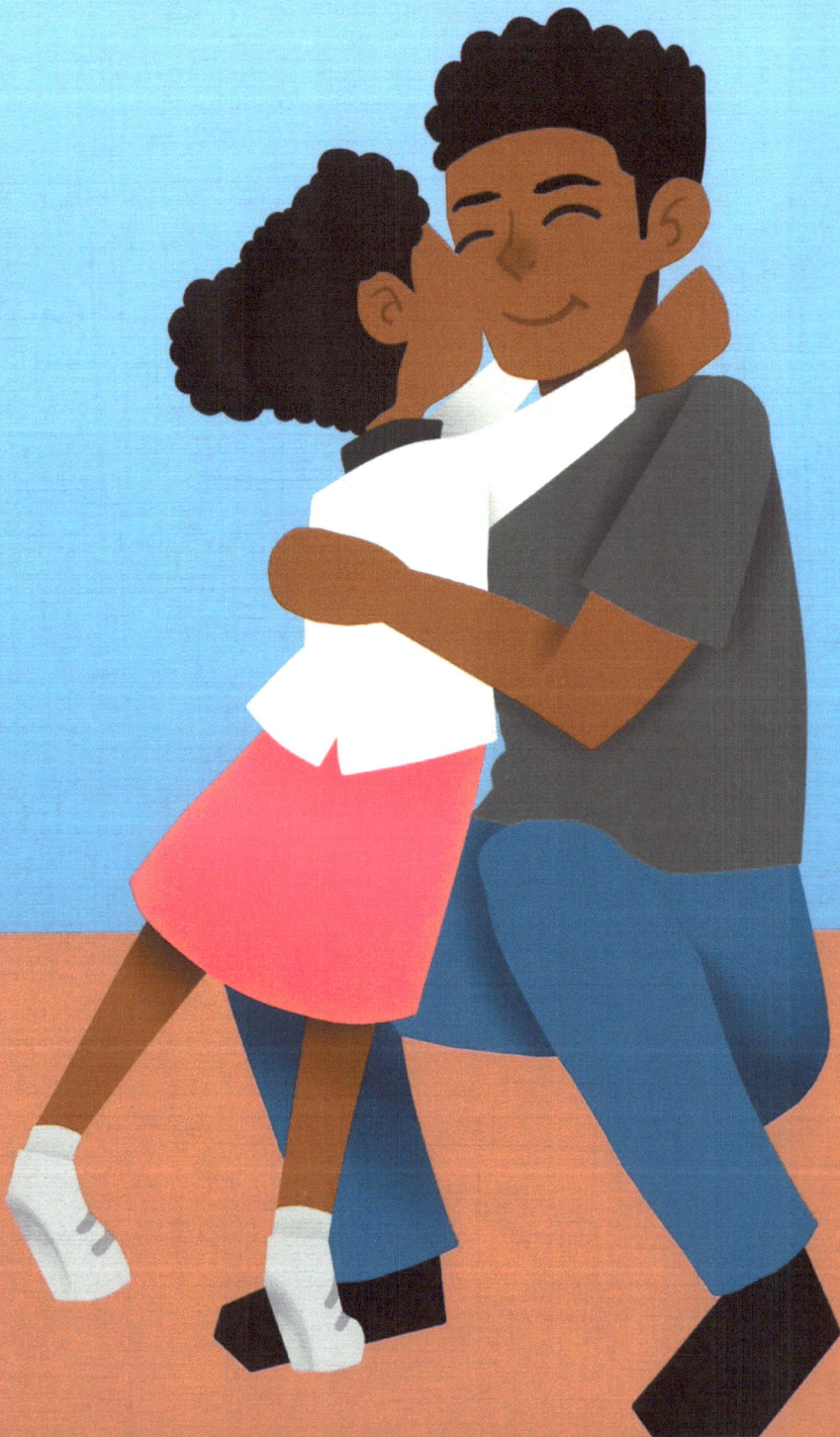

The End.

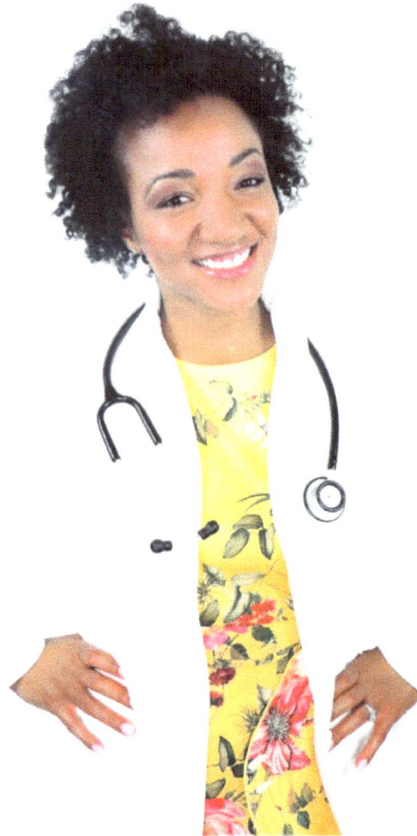

Dr. Cymanthia Connell is a board-certified family doctor born and raised in Montreal, Canada. She is affectionately referred to as "Doctor Cyam" by her family and "Auntie Cyam" by the younger ones including Samia. Dr. Cyam is a proud ambassador for healthy everyday living to prevent illness. She is currently practicing in the Greater Atlanta Area in Georgia.

Stay up to date with Dr. Cyam by visiting www.drcyam.com

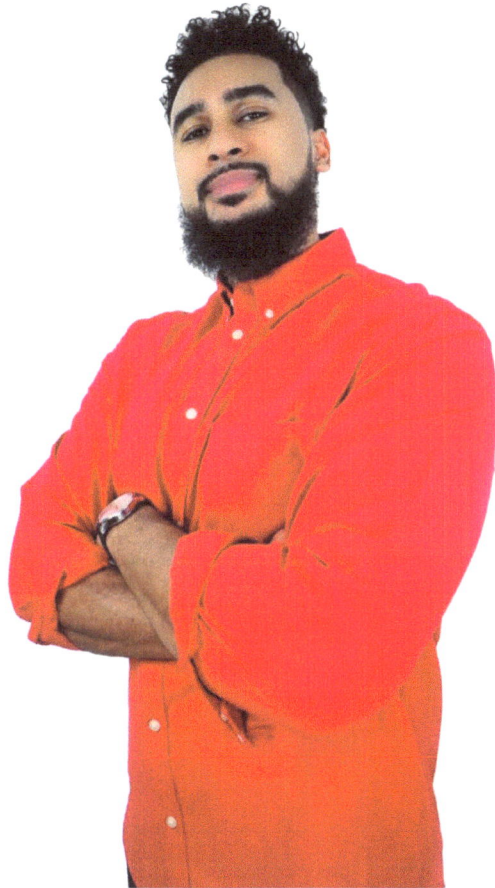

Adam Ali is a full-time online video creator based in Toronto and Atlanta with a passion for telling visual stories. He's excited to incorporate practical life lessons through his daughter's book series. After seeing his daughter's love for reading time, Adam became inspired to write a book with his daughter as the main character. He believes kids at this tender age can absorb some of the best lessons to shape their lives positively. He continues to inspire Samia to provide educational and fun messaging in her online videos and aims to do the same in future books too.

Stay up to date with Adam and Samia Ali on their family Youtube channel:
Youtube.com/TheAlis

www.ingramcontent.com/pod-product-compliance
Lightning Source LLC
Chambersburg PA
CBHW060845270326
41933CB00003B/202